BREASTFEEDING SOLUTIONS

Sexual Intimacy After the Baby Arrives

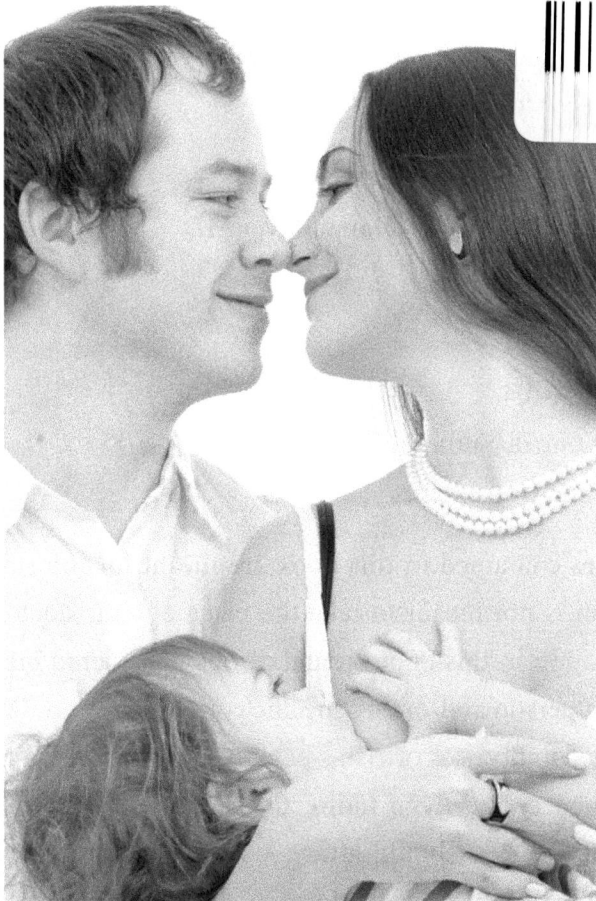

Diana Mayer MD

ISBN: 0-9892294-0-8
ISBN-13: 978-0-9892294-0-1
Library of Congress Control Number: 2013906737
D R Mayer Breastfeeding Consultants

Disclaimer: The pages contained in this book are meant for informational purposes only. This information is not meant to take the place of your doctor or other health provider. The information in this book should not be considered medical advice with respect to any specific person and/or any specific condition. The author, therefore specifically disclaims any liability, loss or risk—personal or otherwise—that is, or may be, incurred as a consequence, directly or indirectly, from use or application of any of the information provided. Readers should always consult their personal physicians and other health providers first regarding all information presented in this book. The author does not endorse or recommend any particular products. Mention of any product is not meant to be a recommendation. Readers should consult a physician in regard to personal use of any product.

ACKNOWLEDGMENTS

Thanks go out to:

Practicing obstetrician and gynecologist Rebecca Cipriano, MD, author of *Pop: Burst the Diet Bubble and Finally Lose Weight,* for her thorough review of this book.

Family medicine and breastfeeding medicine specialist Alicia Dermer, MD IBCLC FABM, for her thorough review of this book and for mentoring me throughout the process of becoming a breastfeeding medicine specialist

Researcher Viola Polomeno, inf./ R.N., Ph. D. for generously allowing me to share her research, techniques and insights with readers

CentraState Medical Center medical librarian, Robin Siegel, whose diligent research has made me and my colleagues look good for many years.

TABLE OF CONTENTS

INTRODUCTION

Congratulations on the birth of your baby! This is a special time in your life. The strong bond that you establish with your baby is both amazing and everlasting. Motherhood changes life in many ways. The baby depends on you. He or she needs your love and attention. Besides the baby, other people are an essential part of your life and still emotionally need you. And—in the midst of your new and demanding life—you have needs too. It is easy to dismiss or put aside your own desires when demands are great and you have so little time. Try not to lose sight of your personal needs. A big challenge will be to balance all parts of your life—including the sexual desires of the two of you as a couple.

For all couples, sex routines change after the baby comes. Regardless of the baby's milk source (mother's milk or infant formula), all couples experience exhaustion and sleep deprivation. This tiredness continues for months after the baby arrives. Some moms may experience low sexual urges (known as low libido) or may feel physical discomfort of their sexual parts during sex. This book covers specific strategies that address these problems.

Nursing moms may run into some unique situations. A few may eject milk from their breasts during sex. Some may have sore or sensitive breasts. Birth control choice also warrants special consideration

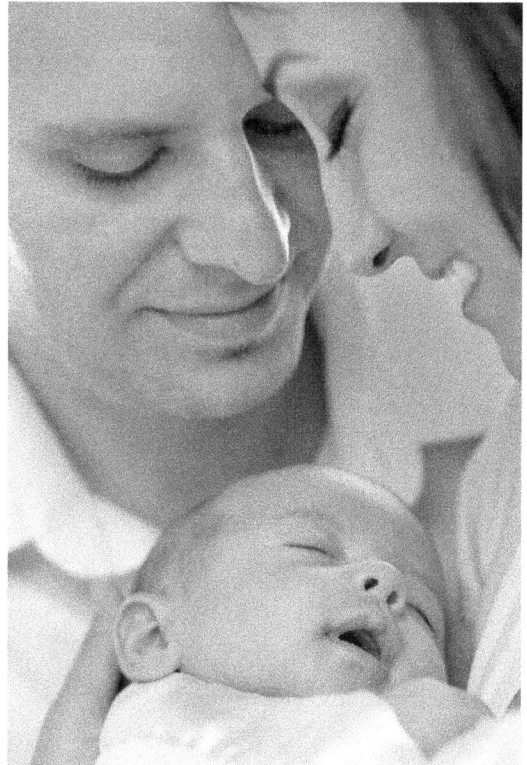

in nursing moms. You will find specific tips and strategies that can help you with these issues.

This book answers questions about your sex life, including special questions you may have as a nursing mother. Hopefully, it will also serve as a launch pad for you to begin a conversation with your doctor or other health care practitioner. Some moms are uncomfortable talking to health care professionals about sex. If you feel this way, realize that they are used to answering a variety of questions about people's sex lives.

It is worth paying attention to your sex life. Remember that your baby benefits when the two of you—as a couple—have a healthy and loving relationship. Your connection as a couple glues your family together as a unit. Each family member benefits from this relationship—including your child.

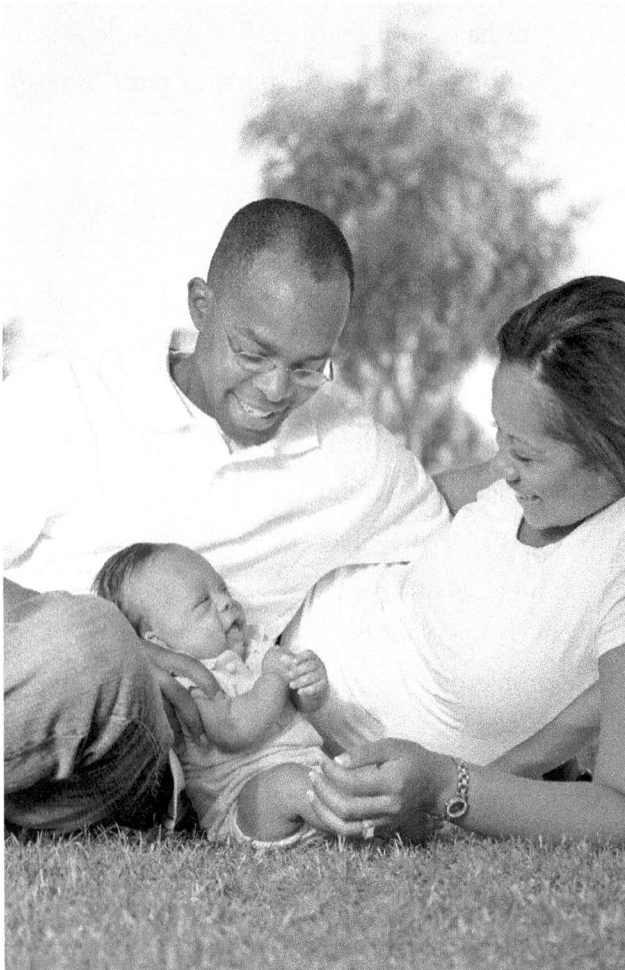

THE LINK BETWEEN MOTHER'S MILK AND GOOD HEALTH:

Why Should I Breastfeed My Baby?

It is clear from research studies that mother's milk increases the chances that your baby will remain healthy and be protected from certain diseases and health conditions. Breastfeeding helps a mom's health as well.

Regarding infants, research shows that the risk of certain infections in infancy and childhood is lower in babies who are fed mother's milk. When infections do occur, they are often milder and of shorter duration. Babies fed mother's milk are more protected from infections, such as the common cold, middle ear infections, and diarrhea disease. Babies are less likely to contract severe bacterial blood infections (known as sepsis), as well as a certain severe intestinal infection that affects some premature babies (known as necrotizing enterocolitis). This is because human milk contains several immune-fighting substances and cells that help fight off infection. Some of these fighters can modify themselves in a way that allows them to target a specific infection.

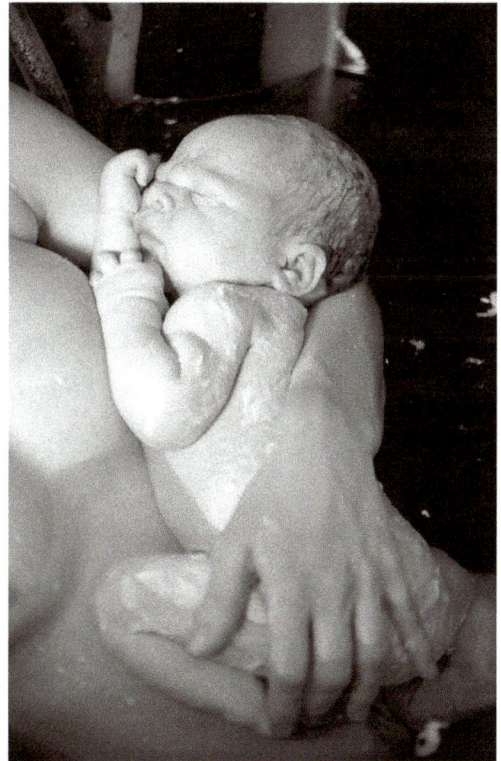

Diabetes, inflammatory bowel disease (e.g., Crohn's disease and ulcerative colitis), asthma, eczema, sudden infant death syndrome (SIDS), and obesity are seen less often in babies who were breastfed when compared to those who were not. Acute lymphocytic leukemia of childhood occurs less often in children who received human milk for at least six months (a 19 percent reduction). There is also some evidence of modest increases in IQ points in those who were fed human milk.

Mothers who have nursed are more protected from breast cancer and ovarian cancer compared to those who have not, especially if the cumulative (number of months breastfeeding all of their children) amount of breastfeeding time is more than twelve months. Type 2 diabetes in later life is also reduced in certain moms who have breastfed. Postpartum depression is seen less often in mothers who breastfeed. Additionally, it may be easier for mothers to lose their pregnancy weight because they burn off an average five hundred calories each day while making milk.

Receiving breastmilk as the only milk source for a minimum of twelve months (and starting baby food at about six months) has a significant impact on the good health outcomes described above for infant and mother. However, continuing beyond twelve months improves some of these health outcomes even more.

COMMON QUESTIONS

What if my breasts are sore?

Some—though not all—nursing moms may feel breast discomfort at some point or another while breastfeeding. Most of the time, it is temporary and goes away. Breasts can be sore or sensitive for a variety of reasons. It is important to figure out whether the soreness is due to a nursing problem or an underlying medical problem.

Some types of breast discomfort are transient. Moms may feel nipple and areolar (the colored part of the breast that surrounds the nipple) discomfort during the first one to two weeks of nursing. Starting from the time of birth, the mother's breast tissue gets pulled in new ways while the baby is suckling. The breast tissue must get used to being stretched, just like muscles must get used to being stretched and pulled for the first couple of weeks after starting a workout routine at the gym. This normal breast tissue stretching should only feel uncomfortable for less than a minute after the baby latches. It should never result in sores, cracks, bleeding, or bruising on the breasts. Stretching discomfort is usually totally gone within a week or two of the infant's birth.

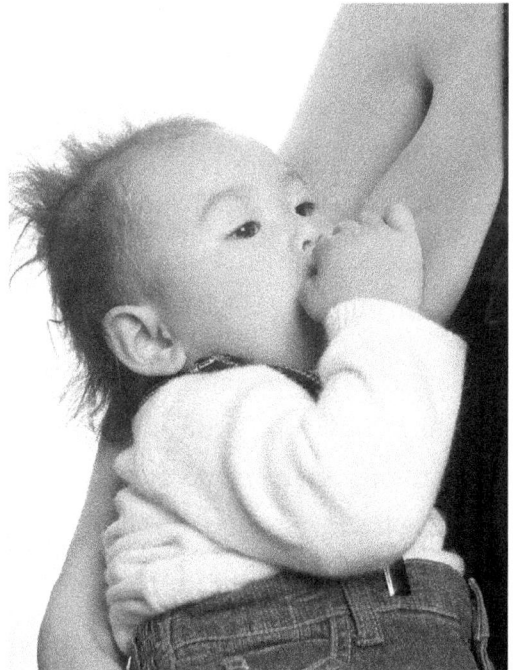

Another kind of temporary breast discomfort is from the normal breast fullness women note around two to four days after birth. This is the time that large amounts of milk fill the breasts in response to normal hormone surges. This phase usually calms down within two to four days. A mother's discomfort is decreased if she directly nurses every time the baby is hungry. Using bottles (or pacifiers) will result in less complete emptying of the breasts, leading to more breast swelling and pain.

A mother can safely take ibuprofen (Advil, Motrin) or acetaminophen (Tylenol) to help relieve some of this breast engorgement discomfort. This will not hurt the baby. Remember that some prescribed pain medications, such as Percocet, already contain acetaminophen. If you have been prescribed a combination pain pill that contains acetaminophen, don't take any extra plain acetaminophen.

While moms are in this phase, many experts recommend applying warm compresses for a few minutes on the breast before a feeding (to increase milk flow) and then cold compresses following the feeding (to decrease inflammation). If your baby has trouble latching deeply due to breast fullness, hand express some milk out of the front part of the breasts (a lactation consultant can teach you how to do this). This softens your breast tissue, allowing easier and deeper latching.

Call your health care provider, as well as a lactation consultant, if you feel breast discomfort throughout the feeding. Call if you have clogged ducts, breast or nipple sores, redness, bruising, or if the nipples turn blue, purple, or white at the tips. Your health provider will rule out any breast conditions, while the lactation consultant will evaluate your baby's latch. Signs of a breast infection, known as mastitis, may include breast pain, along with a hot, sore red area on the breast. Women with mastitis may have achiness, fever, and extreme exhaustion. Any one of these signs may signify the start of a breast infection. Call your health professional right away if any of these signs occur.

Have a lactation consultant and your baby's doctor check your baby's mouth for structural problems. Some of these problems, such as a high, arched roof of the mouth or short tongue, are temporary and responsive to certain interventions. Others, such as a tongue tie, may require a simple office procedure, known as a frenotomy, where the tongue tie tissue is snipped.

What about breast sensitivity and sex? Some—though not all—nursing mothers' breasts may be sensitive to touch, even though no medical reason can be found (Leeman et al. 2012; Polomeno 1999). Partners may need to change the way they touch sensitive breasts. Some mothers may find deep hand massage, nipple pinching/rolling or sucking of the breasts very uncomfortable. However, certain kinds of breast touching can be more comfortable and possibly arousing. One source (Polomeno 1999) suggests that a partner gently hold both breasts in the palms of the hands and slowly sway them from one side to the other in unison. Some mothers experience brief periods of sexual arousal with this maneuver. Regarding breast kissing, light, gentle kissing may be more pleasurable than sucking on the nipples.

Rarely, mothers may have trouble even with light touch. This requires discussion as a couple. If a woman is extremely sensitive to any breast touching during sexual encounters, it may need to be avoided for a period of time. Sensual pleasuring of other body areas would then become the couple's focus.

When can we start having sex again?

Always check with your health care provider for the final okay to begin having sex. He or she will usually recommend that a couple can start having sexual intercourse six weeks after the baby's birth. Sometimes, a doctor or other health care practitioner will give the green light at the four week mark, but always check with him or her first. He or she must make sure that any tears or sutured wounds from childbirth have healed and that the tip of the womb, known as the cervix, is back to normal.

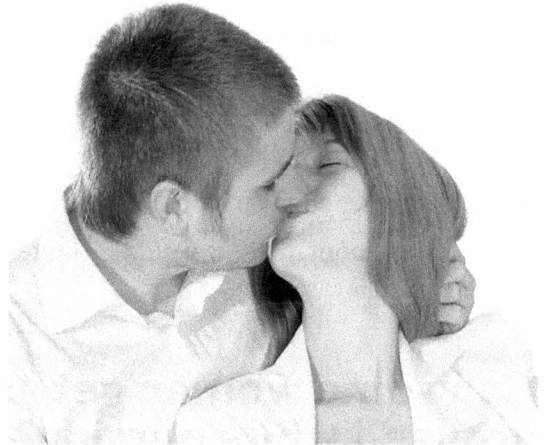

What if I have a milk letdown release during sex?

The love hormone, oxytocin, is released from the brains of both men and women during orgasm. Oxytocin causes the general feeling of well-being and satisfaction associated with orgasm. The mother's brain also secretes oxytocin during nursing, causing the milk letdown response (also known as the milk ejection reflex). This is why for a few women, milk will spurt from the breasts during orgasm. Couples handle this in different ways. Some decide to incorporate the milk ejection into their lovemaking experience.

These couples either don't mind if the letdown happens or view the milk ejection as a turn-on. For other couples, the milk ejection reflex while climaxing feels distracting or undesirable. In this case, the strategies outlined in this section will help.

Some moms press their nipples with their hands in order to control the spurt of milk from their breasts during an orgasm (Reader 2005). Others have a towel nearby that they toss over their breasts while becoming aroused. Some moms create a sensual atmosphere by draping over their breasts a black or red towel (or lace material from the fabric store). However, if it takes too much work to purchase this, just keep life simple and grab the nearest towel.

If you feel nervous about the possibility that your body will eject milk during sex, try wearing a padded nursing bra the first few times you are intimate with your partner. Check the bra pads afterward for milk. Keep in mind that sexy nursing bras are now available—often with matching panties—for those who would like to enhance the atmosphere. Many are lacy and come in a variety of colors. Check a specialty store or use a computer search engine (for instance, search "sexy nursing bras") to locate stores that carry them.

Some couples prefer having sex after the baby has nursed and has fallen asleep. Milk ejection during sex is less likely when the baby has removed a good deal of milk. Using this strategy depends on whether the two of you are willing to plan your time for sex. If you prefer spontaneity, it would be better to use one of the other strategies described in this section.

Can some women get sexually aroused while nursing?

A *few* mothers have reported feeling a sensation similar to—but not exactly like—orgasm while nursing. This is due to contraction of the uterus from oxytocin hormone release. The feeling is usually described as the sense of well-being and satisfaction people feel after orgasm, though genital arousal is usually not involved. Some moms feel awkward and embarrassed about this experience (Von Sydow 1999; Avery et al. 2000). If anything like this has happened to you, it is an unintentional event that is nothing to be ashamed of, like any other physical feeling. One source suggests that uncrossing the legs while nursing may help lower the chances of experiencing this type of sensation (Polomeno 1999).

What if I just don't feel like having sex?

Not wanting sex most or all of the time, also known as low libido, is common in new mothers—and fathers—regardless of how they are feeding their baby (nursing or infant formula feeding). If you have had little or no sexual desire since giving birth, know that it takes at least two to three months following the baby's arrival before most couples begin feeling in the mood. If your sexual urge remains low after this period, there are things that you can try that may help make it better. The first thing to think about is why your sexual urge is low. A low libido can occur for a variety of reasons, as explained below.

STRESS AND EXHAUSTION: WHAT HELPS

All parents experience stress and exhaustion as they meet the needs of the baby and also tend to other aspects of their lives. Some ways to decrease stress or exhaustion may include the following:

- Consider asking for help with daily activities. Fewer daily worries may make you feel more open to having sex. If someone does help out, remember that he or she may not do things exactly the same way as you. Try to let go of the need to have things done precisely as they are usually done.

- Though most of the time you will try to sleep when the baby sleeps, parents report that the best time to have sex is right after the baby falls asleep following nursing. This lowers the risk of infant interruption.

- Don't expect your house to look perfectly tidy. Both of you should keep in mind that a "relaxed you" is more likely to start thinking about sex compared to a "stressed, uptight you." However, if you feel extremely stressed out by living in an untidy house, discuss this. Explain that the messy house prevents you from relaxing and getting in the mood for sex. Discuss that helping you with housework will remove this barrier.

- See the Getting in the Mood section later in this booklet.

POSTPARTUM DEPRESSION

Within two weeks of the baby's arrival, more than 50 percent of moms have bouts of feeling overwhelmed, sad, and tearful regardless of how they have decided to feed the baby. They may have a loss of appetite. They may have trouble sleeping well. This is known as the baby blues. Baby blues stems from expected exhaustion, as well as from the hormonal changes that happen in a woman's body following the baby's birth. Call your health care provider if your feelings are getting worse or if they don't disappear by the time the baby is two weeks old.

If these symptoms don't resolve within two weeks of the baby's birth, postpartum depression may be setting in. These feelings can stay at the same intensity or may get stronger.

Onset of symptoms can vary. Some moms can begin experiencing symptoms of depression shortly after the baby's birth, while symptoms in other moms do not come out until three to four months later.

Postpartum depression symptoms can include:

- feeling sad, anxious, or overwhelmed
- tearful spells
- mood swings
- trouble sleeping
- loss of appetite
- little or no interest in your baby
- thoughts of hurting yourself or hurting the baby

Rarely, mothers will experience postpartum psychosis, which is the most severe type of postpartum depression. Contact your doctor immediately if you have experienced the symptoms below or if somebody has told you that they think you have these symptoms:

- feeling confused
- a sense that someone is trying to hurt you
- intense mood swings
- hearing or seeing things that someone has told you aren't there
- thoughts of hurting yourself or attempts to hurt yourself
- thoughts of hurting your baby or attempts to hurt your baby

Some studies suggest that breastfeeding moms are less likely to experience postpartum depression than mothers who formula feed. It is thought that the frequent release of the milk ejection hormone, oxytocin, helps maintain a general feeling of well-being. However, despite this, some nursing moms may still have postpartum depression.

If you or your family worry that you have postpartum depression, get help. Never keep your sad feelings to yourself! There are steps you can take to help feel better! Call your doctor, a postpartum depression hotline, or a therapist. One national online source is Postpartum Support International (www.postpartum.net). In the US, most states have websites and hotline numbers dedicated to postpartum depression.

If your doctor recommends antidepressant medication, know that several are safe to take while nursing. Some drug information sources for breastfeeding mothers are more reliable than others. While most doctors are aware of the more accurate medication information sources, others may not be. Doctors and other practitioners should use references such as LactMed online (http://toxnet.nlm.nih.gov/cgi-bin/sis/htmlgen?LACT) or Thomas W. Hale's book, *Medications and Mother's Milk*. The Academy of Breastfeeding Medicine, an international physicians' group that is solely dedicated to breastfeeding medicine, publishes a free protocol about antidepressant medication use in nursing mothers. Two medication call centers will take phone calls from health professionals (but not the general public) seeking advice about drug safety in breastfeeding mothers. This includes the Infant Risk Center hotline at Texas Tech University Health Sciences Center (806-352-2519) and the Lactation Studies Center hotline at the University of Rochester (585-275-0088). These call centers are available during daytime weekday hours. It is okay if you ask your health care provider to check a few of these sources.

DOMESTIC (OR RELATIONSHIP) ABUSE

It is very hard to feel like having sex if you are in an abusive relationship. Women may experience physical, psychological, and/or emotional abuse, all of which often get worse during pregnancy and after a baby arrives. If you are in this position, the priority is to keep your baby and yourself safe. In the US, call the National Domestic Violence Hotline at 800-799-7233 (TTY 800-787-3224) or visit their website at www.thehotline.org when you are able to find a safe time and place to do so. In addition to calling a hotline, talk to your health care provider, a therapist, or religious leader that you trust.

PELVIC PAIN

There are many reasons for pelvic pain following childbirth. Most commonly, pelvic discomfort is transient after a baby's delivery. This kind of pain gradually goes away over several weeks. However, pain that worsens or continues may be due to other problems. If you are experiencing pelvic pain, it is important to see your health care provider. He or she will help you identify the source of your discomfort. Recommendations and treatment will depend on the underlying cause of the pain. This may possibly include the use of certain over-the-counter products, prescription medication, physical therapy, or, in very rare circumstances, surgical correction.

If your health care provider prescribes physical therapy, he or she will likely recommend physical therapists (PTs) in your community who are knowledgeable about women's health problems and pelvic pain. Additionally, physical therapy associations may point you to therapists who have a special interest in this area. In the US, the American Physical Therapy Association website (www.apta.org) includes a PT finder page that helps patients identify therapists who focus on these problems. (Choose the women's health check box first. Descriptions of specific services, such as physical therapy for pelvic pain, are listed under certain therapist's names.)

Common sources of pelvic pain are listed in the sections below.

EPISIOTOMY SITE SENSITIVITY

Some women don't want to have sex because their episiotomy scar causes discomfort. If you suspect that painful sex may be due to an episiotomy scar, have your health care provider check this out. If he or she suspects that this is where your pain is coming from, he or she will talk about different options that might help you feel more comfortable during sex. Options include generous use of lubricants (see the next section) or physical therapy to loosen the scar and strengthen pelvic muscles. Sometimes, if discomfort does not improve, surgical revision of the scar is necessary.

VAGINAL DRYNESS

Hormonal changes may result in vaginal dryness in some nursing mothers (Avery et al. 2000). Low lubrication is due to decreased levels of the female hormone, estrogen. The good news is that easily accessible remedies exist that can significantly improve vaginal dryness.

Signs of low natural vaginal lubrication include discomfort, scant bleeding (from irritation), and burning/itching during or after sex. Keep in mind that some of these complaints can also be observed when women have vaginal yeast infections. Health care providers will help sort this out and recommend the right treatment.

Product Categories

If your symptoms are due to vaginal dryness, sex can become more pleasurable with the use of personal lubricants and long-lasting vaginal moisturizers. Several kinds are available (without a prescription) to help fix this problem. Long-lasting vaginal moisturizers are used to keep the vagina moist throughout the day and night. Used on a routine basis, long-lasting vaginal moisturizers are usually inserted in the vagina, via a slender applicator, every three days (Andelloux, 2011; Herbenick, D., et al. 2009). The frequency of insertion varies from product to product, though many products permit use as frequently as once a day. Some examples include Replens and Luvena.

Personal lubricants are used with sexual activity, including foreplay and intercourse (Andelloux, 2011; Herbenick, D., et al. 2009). Some common lubricants are Astroglide Gel, K-Y Jelly, and Liquid Silk. Many other brands, including generic lubricants, are available as well.

Some women use both long-lasting vaginal moisturizers (for overall long-lasting vaginal tissue moisturizing) and personal lubricants (during sexual activity). It is usually okay to use both kinds of products. Call your health practitioner for a recommendation, and follow package recommendations.

Ingredients

A few people may experience side effects from ingredients in these products. It is prudent to test topical products on a small area of your skin (your partner too) for a couple of days before use, because some people can develop a rash. This is especially true with products containing parabens (also listed in the product's ingredient list as methylparaben, propylparaben, or butylparaben). Parabens are a group of preservatives that extend product shelf life. Up to 20 percent of people develop a skin reaction to these products (Andelloux, 2011; Herbenick, D., et al. 2009). Several manufacturers make paraben-free products for those with this sensitivity (for instance, Glycerin & Paraben-Free Astroglide, Astroglide Natural, Slippery Stuff Paraben-Free, and Wet Ecstasy Silicone, to name just a few). Some long-lasting vaginal moisturizers are paraben-free as well (e.g., Luvena Prebiotic Vaginal Moisturizer).

Glycerin is another ingredient that is added to most lubricants because it improves the taste. Lubricants without glycerin can sometimes taste bitter. While most women tolerate lubricants with glycerin very well, a glycerin-containing product would not be a good choice for women who are prone to vaginal yeast infections (Andelloux, 2011; Herbenick, D., et al. 2009). Several glycerin-free lubricants are available (for instance, Glycerin & Paraben Free Astroglide, Astroglide Natural, Blossom Organics Moisturizing Lubricant, Pink Silicone Lubricant for Women, Babeland BabeLube, and Good Clean Love Lubricant). For vegans, Babeland BabeLube states that the product is vegan and animal cruelty-free. Good Clean Love is also a vegan product. Some long-lasting vaginal moisturizers, such as Luvena Prebiotic Vaginal Moisturizer, are glycerin-free.

Types of Personal Lubricants

Types of personal lubricants include water-based, silicone-based, petroleum-based, and natural oil-based products. Water-based lubricants are most often recommended because they are least likely to break down condoms. They are also less expensive and easier to find. Applying the lubricant on the outside female parts (the vulva and clitoris, around/over the entrance of your vagina), as well as on the partner's genitals, will help make sex more comfortable and enjoyable. Frequent application may be needed because water-based lubricants can dry up quickly. Always check the manufacturer's instructions before application (Andelloux, 2011; Herbenick, D., et al. 2009). Some examples of water-based lubricants are K-Y Jelly, Astroglide Gel, and Wet Original Gel. Liquid Silk is also water-based, though a small amount of added silicone helps this product last longer, according to the manufacturer.

Silicone lubricants may be helpful for people with sensitive skin. The major advantage is that they last longer during sexual encounters than the water-based products. They also work well for sexual encounters in water environments (bathtubs, etc). Though people really like these products, they tend to cost more, they are harder to remove from skin, and they can stain sheets. Some of these products may have an undesirable taste. They are generally compatible with condom use, but check package instructions (Andelloux, 2011; Herbenick, D., et al. 2009). Some examples of silicone lubricants include Wet Platinum, K-Y Intrigue, Astroglide X Premium Silicone, and Pink Silicone Lubricant for Women.

Petroleum-based lubricants (Vaseline, mineral oil) are often irritating to genital tissue. Natural oil-based lubricants (vegetable oil, olive oil) may also irritate genital tissue. Both can break down condoms and stain sheets (Andelloux, 2011; Herbenick, D., et al. 2009).

Shopping for Products

Personal lubricants and long-lasting vaginal moisturizers can be purchased online or at a physical store (usually a drugstore). Brand availability varies from one store to the next. For this reason, it is important to identify whether a product is a long-lasting vaginal moisturizer or personal lubricant by inspecting the package. If you intend on avoiding certain ingredients, get used to reading the ingredient section of the package. Look for words that include terms such as paraben (methylparaben, propylparaben, or butylparaben) or glycerin. Most packages will point out if the product is free of certain products.

Other Products

Use of prescription topical estrogen (in the form of either a cream, an insertable vaginal ring or insertable vaginal tablet) is sometimes recommended by health care practitioners, though its use by breastfeeding mothers is somewhat controversial. While some experts believe that topical application of estrogen on a woman's genital area is unlikely to decrease milk volume, others recommend its use only after other methods have failed. Topical estrogen products are largely prescribed for mothers of infants who are at least six months old. However, some mothers of younger infants have used these products very successfully. If you do use it, keep close track of the baby's urine and bowel movement frequency, as well as his or her weight.

Other Tips

Brief sensual activities at other points in the day can build up a sense of anticipation, increasing natural vaginal lubrication. An increase in sexual interest and arousal is associated with activities such as sharing of sexual fantasies, playful flirting and spontaneous quick kisses or hugs at other points in the day. The next section of this book (Getting in the Mood) explores this in more detail.

Additionally, engaging in longer foreplay prior to intercourse usually increases natural vaginal lubrication.

- **Please note:** Because product ingredients may be changed over time, always check product ingredients on the package or check with the manufacturer. Check with your health-care provider as well.

GETTING IN THE MOOD

ntimacy is the process of connecting with one another in a way that creates a close, warm, and deep relationship. Couples may experience intimacy on physical, psychological, emotional, and spiritual levels. Physical intimacy is more likely to be achieved if the other intimacy types are also a part of the relationship. Though there is no proven method that guarantees sexual intimacy, creating certain conditions in your environment, as well as in your relationship, can set the stage for desire.

Though it may be hard to get in the mood for sex when you're exhausted or busy, the following are some ways to spice up your love life.

Optimize opportunities and surroundings

- A good time to have sex is when the baby is napping. However, if a young baby is awake, quiet, and in a safe place (such as a bassinet, infant swing, or playpen) and within the same room as the two of you, there is nothing wrong with some impromptu sex. A young baby is not going to be aware of your sexual encounters (on the other hand, an older infant or your toddler might).

- Don't assume that the only time to have sex is after the baby is sleeping at night. While nighttime may be the best time for some couples, consider other parts of the day. Some couples experiment with sex in the early morning or during the baby's afternoon naptimes.

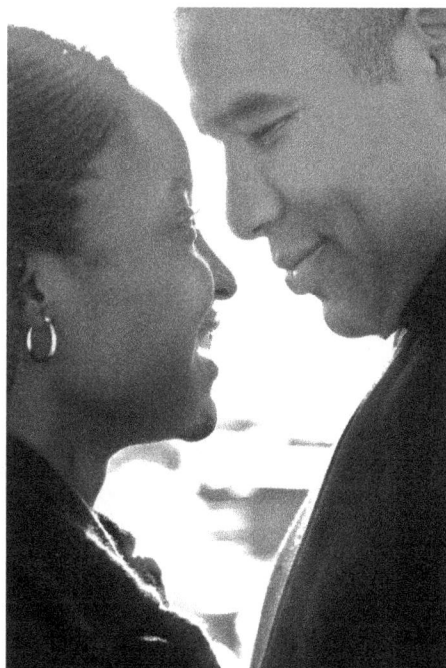

- Think beyond the bedroom. Exhausted couples may avoid having sex on their bed because it makes them feel too sleepy, opting instead for sex in other areas of the home. Have sex in places that are most convenient for the two of you, not just your bed. Some couples report having sex in their parked vehicle (engine off) located in the driveway or garage while their young baby is fast asleep in a car seat.

Physical closeness

- Couples who hug and hold each other frequently may begin feeling more in the mood for sex, even if either person did not feel in the mood at first. Researchers have discovered that holding and hugging each other for at least twenty to thirty seconds causes the release of the love hormone, oxytocin (Grewen 2005; Light et al. 2005).

- Playful actions, including spontaneous hugs, a surprise kiss, pats on the rear end, etc., can set the stage for more intense foreplay later on

- Some women report that, in the post-baby period, sexual desire may start in the middle of the lovemaking process rather than at the beginning. It is possible that even if you are not initially in the mood for sex on first approach, kissing and touching may bring those forgotten sexy feelings back.

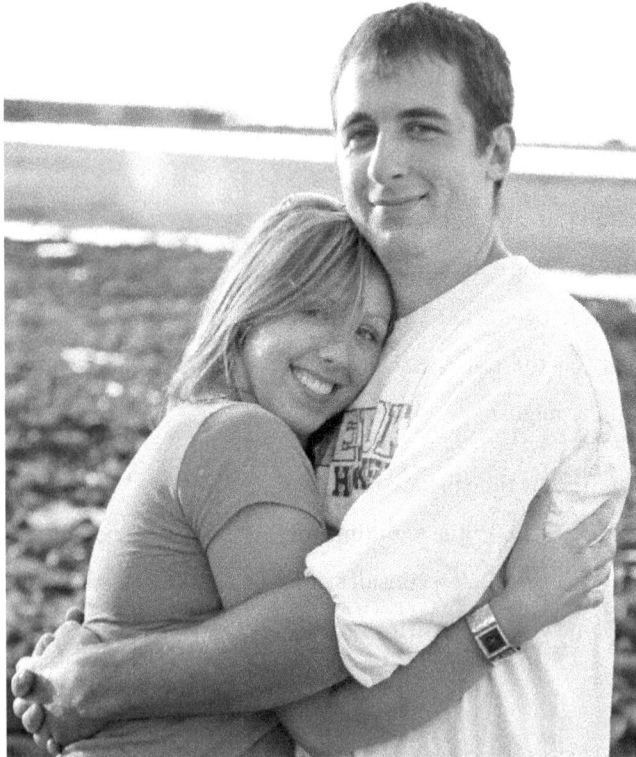

- Couples may be satisfied enough most of the time with quick sexual encounters that don't necessarily end with intercourse.

- Some couples have a discussion—in a nonjudgmental manner—acknowledging that the one with greater sexual urges may have a need to be pleasured (or to masturbate) during the sexual awakening process of the other partner (Von Sydow 2002; also see the "Steps toward building intimacy" below). Consider gently and sensitively discussing the topic. Try to understand this need.

Psychological intimacy: anticipation

- Set the stage by building up excitement. Chat early in the day about what you want to do with each other, or mention a fantasy that has been a turn-on for both of you in the past (Leitenberg et al. 1995). Over the course of the day, occasionally bring up a part of the fantasy.

- Compliments (such as, "You look hot in those jeans," or "That blouse looks fantastic on you," etc.) help each partner feel valued and appreciated. This builds confidence and makes couples more receptive to physical closeness.

- Find ways to flirt either in person, through phone calls, by leaving a note, ect.

- Read a steamy fantasy passage from a book or an article to each other.

Spiritual and emotional intimacy

Keeping your spirit up is important. Your spirit impacts your sense of well-being. Since there is little time to do big things for yourself, commit to at least doing little things during the day. Try some of the following:

- If you used to wear makeup and haven't lately, put some on each morning (even if you don't plan on going anywhere). You will be surprised at what a pick-me-up applying even a small amount of makeup can be. If you never wore makeup in the past, choose something else that makes you feel pretty, such as styling your hair or wearing jewelry.

- If you have been living in sweat pants, it's time to wear something else. The same goes for T-shirts or sweatshirts. Wearing clothes with a little more style-including those types you used to wear before pregnancy-will help energize you.

- Consider abandoning the big, roomy, cotton panties. Routinely wear prettier or sexier ones. This may help you get back in touch with your sensual self (even if you may not always feel that way these days).

- Get outside. If someone else is around to watch the baby, sit in the backyard or go for a ten-minute walk by yourself. Or take the baby with you. Exposure to UV light from the sun is scientifically known to help lift people emotionally.

- Ask a friend to come over for a visit, or visit that friend with the baby. Maintaining a support system through friendship serves as a reminder that people love and care about you. Staying connected is uplifting.

- Join a "mommy and me" or breastfeeding support group. Knowing other people who are going through the same joys and challenges as you is helpful in many ways. Mothers who belong to these kind of support groups share ideas and resources. They problem-solve. They laugh. Some may begin planning play dates outside the support group. Some form long-lasting friendships.

- The emotional connection between the two of you can get lost in all of the parenthood chaos. Remember to say, "I love you." Reminisce about the good old days when you first met and fell in love. Staying connected on an emotional level is important in sustaining your relationship in the long run. This bond may also help the physical connections flow more naturally.

- Consider praying or meditating—even if it is only for sixty seconds. Some women do this while nursing the baby. Others briefly pray or meditate as a couple. Giving yourself a spiritual time-out from the daily humdrum may help boost you up emotionally.

Understanding her needs

Partners should check the table below for some additional ways to stay connected.

Some Ways to Stay Connected with Her

- Tell her that she looks beautiful when she is nursing the baby.

- Tell her that you love her.

- Compliments help reassure her that you continue to find her attractive.

- Bring her something to drink or eat.

- Help with chores.

- Help with baby care between nursing.

- Offer a back scratch or shoulder massage.

- Humor and playful teasing may lighten both of your moods.

- She may need reassurance that the normal changes in her body (wider hips, changes in the shape of her belly, weight gain) from the pregnancy are not unappealing to you. If she tells you that she feels self-conscious, be aware that many women have these views of their bodies after the baby has arrived. These changes are normal following pregnancy. Tell her that you think she is very sexy and irresistible.

- Together discuss the suggestions listed in the Getting in the Mood section above.

- If you both are spiritual people by nature, tap into it together—even if it is only for sixty seconds (pray, meditate).

If you still have trouble getting in the mood, you may just need more time to adjust to life after baby. After all, life is very hectic for both of you. In general, the chaos of parenthood gets somewhat better as the baby gets older. But be reassured: over time, many couples begin experiencing less pressure and develop more sexual interest.

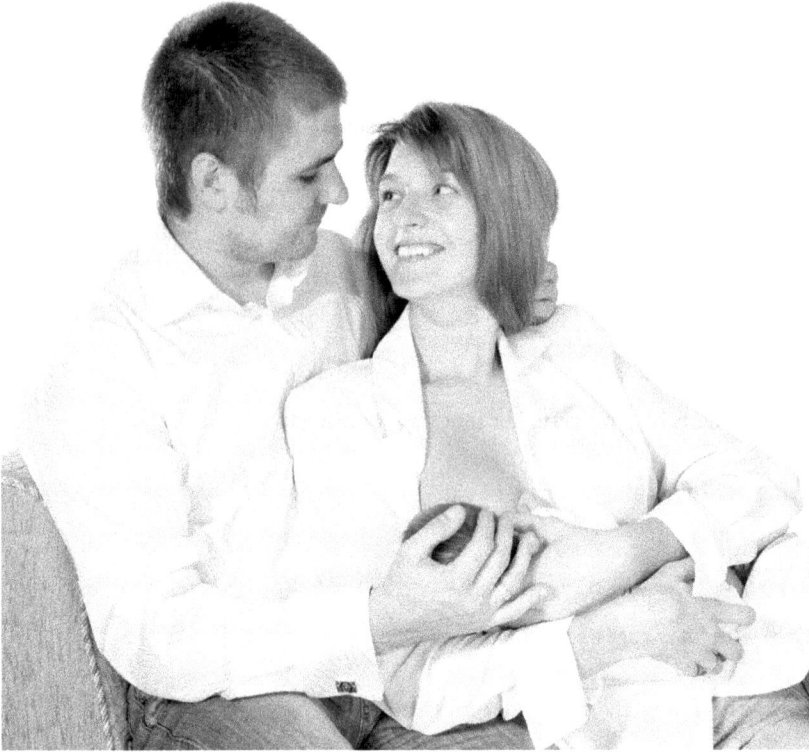

Though there is no guaranteed way to jumpstart one's sex life, some people may find the steps leading toward sexual reawakening, described below, useful. If none of the strategies described in this section have helped and you are very concerned about your relationship, talk to your health care provider or a sex therapist. A good resource is The American Association of Sexuality Educators, Counselors and Therapists (www.aasect. org/directory.asp).

Steps leading toward sexual reawakening

Trying to just snap out of your low libido (sexual urge) rarely works. Instead, think about the underlying reasons that you don't feel like having sex (see above). See your physician or other health care practitioner for a checkup. Along with considering some of the strategies already discussed, one article in the *Journal of Perinatal Education* (Polomeno 1999) describes ways that women may reawaken their sexual selves. This method includes four steps that increase intimacy over time. In this process, couples gradually share both their physical and emotional selves. Advancement from one step to the next may take from a few days to up to two months. The pace depends on what is mutually agreeable by the couple.

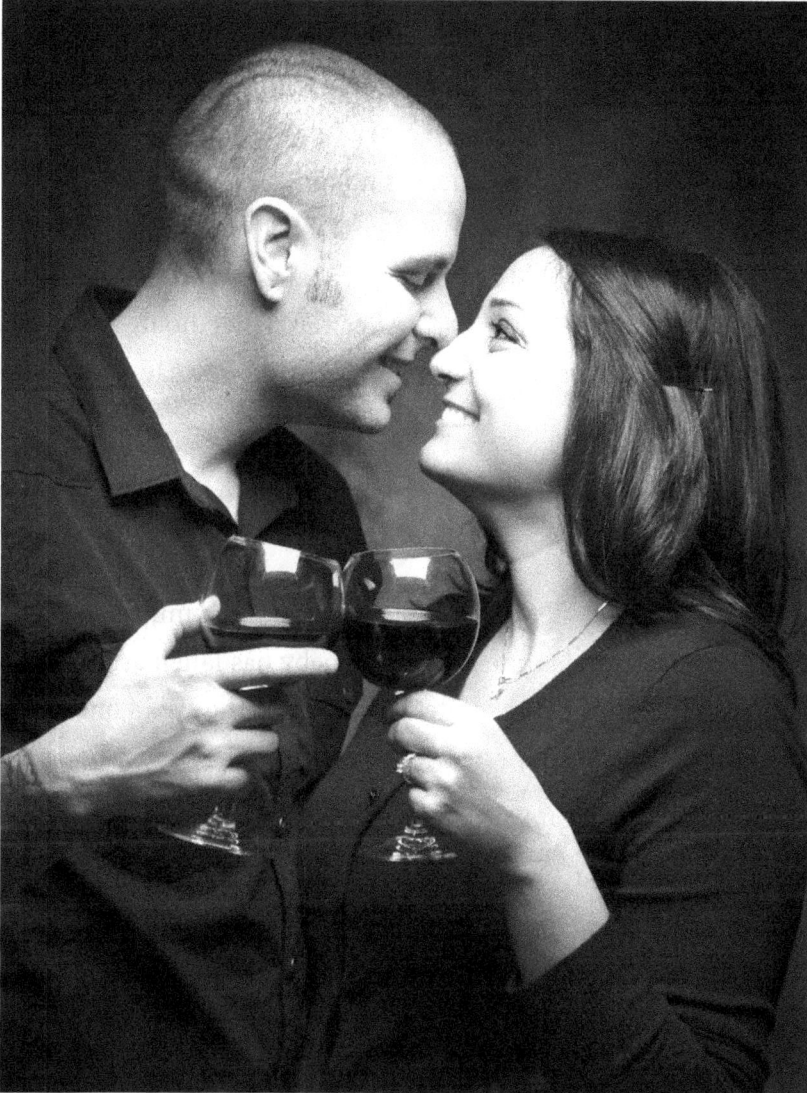

If this approach is not helpful, consult a couple's therapist, and return to your health care provider to check whether further medical intervention is needed.

Below is a general summary from this article (with a few added comments from this author).

Starting off the process

The couple starts off the sexual reawakening process by carving out time to do something together without the baby (go to www.breastfeedingheadquarters.com for Rules for Drinking Alcohol and a tip sheet on Getting Milk out of the Breasts using a breast pump). This may mean dining out or simply going for a brief walk. Once back at home, they hold one another or lightly touch each other. Light touch includes using fingers and/or a feather on one another's bodies. There is no touching of genitals at this point. The author suggests that couples may consider taking a bath or shower together (although you should recognize that it would require a great amount of restraint to refrain from prematurely jumping to the other steps!). Afterward, they hold one another without speaking for ten minutes. After the ten minutes is up, they say a few positive words about their bond to each other.

Following this first encounter, they then proceed to the advice in Step 1.

STEP 1: NONSEXUAL TOUCH.

While working within this step, the couple carves out ten minutes each day in order to lie together. The ideal couple time is after the baby has fallen asleep following nursing (though infant napping is not absolutely necessary). They hold one another without speaking for ten minutes. After the ten minutes is up, they say a few positive words about their bond to each other.

Additionally, hugging and holding each other occasionally during the day is an important part of step 1 (remember that long hugs help release the love hormone, oxytocin). (Grewen 2005).The couple may also carve out extra time for lightly touching each other's skin or bathing/showering together (as described above). Genital touching is avoided while in this step. This takes the pressure off the person who is undergoing sexual reawakening, allowing her room to comfortably move forward through this process (Polomeno 1999; Reader 2005).

STEP 2: NONSEXUAL MASSAGE.

Ideally, the mother nurses the baby first so that the couple will have some time alone with each other while the baby is sleeping (though this is not absolutely necessary).

The couple gives one another a daily massage. The mother receives her massage first. Breasts and genitals are avoided. The couple then holds one another for ten minutes in silence. Following this silence, they say a few positive words about their bond to one another.

STEP 3: EROTIC MASSAGE.

Ideally, the mother nurses the baby first so that the couple will have some time alone together while the baby is sleeping.

While in this step, couples massage one another's bodies, gradually leading toward genital massage. The breasts may or may not be included, depending on how sensitive the nursing woman's breasts are to touch (see section above on touch techniques that women who nurse particularly like). The couple does not have intercourse in Step 3. However, they may include oral-genital pleasuring and use mechanical devices if it is *mutually* comfortable and agreeable. Communicating with each other is emphasized. This might include expressing what feels good, as well as what pressure (harder or softer) or pace (faster or slower) is pleasurable. The couple is encouraged to play music in the background, use oils or creams on one another's bodies, and play out fantasies. They then hold one another for ten minutes in silence. Following this silence, they say a few positive words about their bond to one another. This part of the step is just as important as the physical aspect because the emotional comfort that it promotes helps the couple move closer toward the final step.

STEP 4: MASSAGE AND INTERCOURSE.

Ideally, the mother nurses the baby first so that the couple will have some time with each other while the baby is sleeping.

If a couple wants to know if intercourse will be physically comfortable, the mother does very *gentle* perineal massage (massaging the outside parts of her genitals away and toward her vaginal opening) for one to two minutes followed by insertion of her thumb into her vagina. This gets her skin used to being stretched. Generous use of lubricant is encouraged (see the above section on lubrication). If she does not experience pain during insertion of her thumb, the chances are good that intercourse will be comfortable. If she experiences discomfort, then for the next few days, she should continue the gentle perineal massage followed by thumb insertion into the vagina. This will help her tissue get used to stretching. Once she is pain-free upon thumb insertion, she has her partner *gently* perform the perineal massage followed by the thumb insertion into the vagina. If there is no pain, then intercourse will *likely* feel comfortable.

If anticipation is a turn-on, playful sexual suggestions (or recalling portions of a favorite past sexual fantasy) earlier in the day may set the stage and build excitement.

Some women find that the "on top" sexual intercourse position (also known as the "female dominant" or "woman on top" position) helps maximize comfort during the first few encounters (Reader 2005; Lentz et al. 2012, 157). This position allows her to gauge penile pressure or adjust the pace while having intercourse. Some experts suggest that the "on top" position may particularly help her achieve orgasm, especially if she leans somewhat forward and over her partner (Reader 2005). The "side by side" sexual position is also known to maximize comfort during intercourse (Reader 2005; Lentz et al. 2012, 157). While many couples may find these sexual positions ideal to start with, ultimately couples should choose any mutually desired position.

Couples start their session by massaging one another's bodies, gradually leading toward genital massage. Again, the breasts may or may not be included, depending on how sensitive the nursing woman's breasts are to touch (see section above on touch techniques that women who nurse particularly like). They may lightly touch one another's skin with their fingers or by using a feather. The couple is encouraged to play music in the background, use oils or creams on one another's bodies, and play out fantasies. The couple may include oral-genital pleasuring and use mechanical devices if it is *mutually* comfortable and agreeable. Genital massage eventually leads toward intercourse. Generous use of lubricant on the couple's genitals is encouraged (see above discussion of lubricants). Reapply the lubricant if it starts to dry up. Following intercourse, the couple lies together while holding one another in silence for ten minutes. Then they say a few positive words about their bond to one another. Remember that holding each other and communication following the ten minutes of quiet time are very important components of this step. Both promote closeness as a couple and enhance physical intimacy going forward.

CONTRACEPTION: SPECIAL CONSIDERATIONS IN BREASTFEEDING MOTHERS

Several birth control methods are available to nursing mothers. If you are in need of contraception, discuss and weigh your options with your health care provider. Additionally, the American College of Obstetricians and Gynecologists (www.acog.org) and the Centers for Disease Control and Prevention (go to contraception page at the CDC website, www.cdc.gov) web sites describe contraceptive options. The CDC website includes useful information on failure rates of each birth control method.

Barrier methods

These include condoms, cervical caps, sponges, and spermicides. All are compatible with nursing.

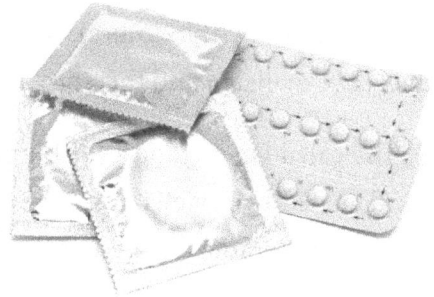

Natural family planning methods

There are two general natural family planning method categories: the lactational amenorrhea method (LAM) and fertility awareness methods (FAM). LAM works by preventing egg release from the ovary (ovulation). Fertility awareness methods require avoidance of sexual intercourse during the fertile portion of a woman's reproductive cycle. This fertile time period is determined by detecting certain body changes. Typical use of the fertility awareness methods enables couples to avoid pregnancy approximately 76% of the time. The lactational amenorrhea method has a success rate of 98% when used properly.

The four types of fertility awareness methods include: basal body temperature, ovulation/cervical mucus, sympatothermal, and calendar methods. The American College of Obstetrics and Gynecology website includes information on how to determine particular fertile periods of the reproductive cycle for each of these fertility awareness methods.

Women who use the basal body temperature method detect ovulation (egg release) by charting body temperature every morning before getting out of bed. A subtle increase in body temperature represents the likely time when ovulation has occurred.

The ovulation/cervical mucus method depends on a women's ability to detect changes in cervix secretions that are present in the vagina (the cervix is the tip of the uterus which is found at the top of a woman's vagina).These secretions become thin and slippery just before the release of an egg from the ovary and remain this way for a few days after ovulation has occurred.

The sympatothermal method combines components of the basal body temperature and the ovulation/cervical mucus methods plus other signs such as abdominal cramping and spotting (if it occurs). All of these signs help women detect the most likely time they have ovulated and therefore know when to avoid sexual intercourse.

The calendar method is also known as the rhythm method. The period of fertility is calculated by reviewing six months of menstrual cycle data and then using certain rules to determine the first and last days of likely fertility. The American College of Obstetrics and Gynecology website gives details on how to determine the fertile phase of a women's cycle (www.acog.org) using this method.

The lactational amenorrhea method (LAM) prevents egg release from the ovaries by controlling an internal hormonal state through consistent breastfeeding and nipple stimulation. It is 98 percent effective as long as three criteria are met: (1) the baby must be less than six months old, (2) the baby cannot receive infant formula or baby food, and breastfeeds should not be delayed with pacifiers or other methods, and (3) the mother has not had her period. As long as all three criteria hold true there should be no need for any hormonal birth control method. However, to cover the 1–2 percent chance of pregnancy with LAM, condoms or diaphragms may be used. Additionally, the American College of Obstetrics and Gynecology website advises that the time interval between breastfeeding times should not be more than every four hours during the day or every six hours at night. This is because an adequate amount of nipple stimulation is needed to prevent egg release from the ovaries

Hormonal contraceptives

Hormonal contraceptives are available as oral medications ("the pill"), injections, or implants. They may contain progesterone or a combination of estrogen and progesterone. These medications are considered compatible with breastfeeding and will not harm the infant. However, in some women, products containing estrogen may significantly decrease the amount of milk made by the breasts. For this reason, progesterone-only products are preferred.

Hormonal contraception should not be introduced until the infant is six weeks of age. This is the time when breastfeeding generally is well established, decreasing the chances of low milk supply. Condoms should be used as backup birth control until oral contraception is considered fully in effect by your health care provider.

Though progesterone-only products are generally recommended over estrogen-containing products, a *few* women may still experience a decrease in milk supply with progesterone-only products. For this reason, Depo-Provera injections (which contain progesterone in the form of a shot that lasts for months) should be considered with caution. This is because the hormones cannot be removed from the body once injected if a milk supply issue occurs. Progesterone implants are another option. While implants can be removed if milk supply problems develop, these devices are a very costly form of contraceptive and are not usually covered by insurance. If used, the risk of potentially needing to remove the implant due to lowered milk volume should be discussed ahead of time.

Intrauterine devices (IUDs)

These devices, including the copper IUD and the progesterone IUD, are compatible with breastfeeding.

Surgical sterilization

This includes male vasectomy and, in females, traditional tubal ligation or hysteroscopic tubal interruption. These forms of contraception are meant for people who are sure that they never want to conceive in the future. Surgical sterilization does not interfere with nursing.

Breastfeeding mothers undergoing a sterilization procedure should either nurse or pump their breasts just prior to the procedure in order to prevent breast discomfort and duct clogging. If general or IV anesthesia is given, a mother can nurse her infant as soon as she regains consciousness and is alert. No "pumping and dumping" of milk is needed. Mothers can safely take acetaminophen (Tylenol) and ibuprofen (Motrin, Advil) for pain as long as it is cleared by their physicians. These medications will not harm the baby. Nursing using the football hold or a side lying position will help avoid any additional abdominal discomfort.

CONCLUSION

Even though life with a baby gets chaotic, there is a path to becoming more intimate with your partner again. This book has described some of the common obstacles that may stand in the way of getting and staying close, as well as the strategies that have helped couples work though them.

Working on your relationship is a worthwhile effort. It will lead to a more content life as a couple. The strong bond between the two of you will strengthen your family and therefore benefit your child in the long run.

May you both enjoy your relationship as a couple and enjoy your new life as parents as well.

RESOURCES

American Academy of Pediatrics breastfeeding website
www2.aap.org/breastfeeding

American College of Obstetricians and Gynecologists
www.acog.org

American Physical Therapy Association website
www.apta.org

Breastfeeding Headquarters
www.breastfeedingheadquarters.com

Centers for Disease Control and Prevention breastfeeding website
www.cdc.gov/breastfeeding

International Society for Sexual Medicine
www.issm.info

International Society for the Study of Women's Sexual Health
www.isswsh.org

Le Leche League International
www.LLLI.org

National Domestic Violence Hotline
www.thehotline.org
(800)779-SAFE [TTY (800)787-3224]

Postpartum Support International
www.postpartum.net

The American Association of Marriage and Family Therapy
www.aamft.org

The American Association of Sexuality Educators, Counselors and Therapists directory
www.aasect.org/directory.asp

The American Board of Sexology
www.americanboardofsexology.com

REFERENCES

American Academy of Pediatrics Section on Breastfeeding. 2012. "Breastfeeding and the use of human milk." *Pediatrics* 129: 598–601.

American College of Obstetricians and Gynecologists www.acog.org

Andelloux, M. 2011. "Products for Sexual Lubrication." *Nursing for Women's Health* 15 (3): 253–257.

Avery, M., et al. 2000. "The Experience of Sexuality During Breastfeeding Among Primiparous Women." *Journal of Midwifery Women's Health* 45: 227–237.

Beral, V, and Reeves, G. July 20, 2002. "Breast cancer and breastfeeding: collaborative reanalysis of individual data from 47 epidemiological studies in 30 countries, including 50,302 women with breast cancer and 96,973 women without the disease." *Lancet* 360 (9328): 187–195.

Convery, K., et al. 2009. "Sexuality and Breastfeeding: What do you Know?" *MCN* 34 (4): 219–223.

Danforth, K. N., Twroger, S. S., Height, J. L., Colditz, G. A., and Hankinson, S. E. 2007. "Breastfeeding and risk of ovarian cancer in two prospective cohorts." *Cancer Causes & Control* 18 (5): 517–523.

Ellis, B., et al. 1990. "Sex Differences in Sexual Fantasy: An Evolutionary Psychological Approach." *The Journal of Sexual Research* 27 (4): 527–555.

Grewen, K. 2005. "Effects of Partner Support on Resting Oxytocin, Cortisol, Norepinephrine and Blood Pressure Before and After Warm Partner Contact." *Psychosomatic Medicine* 67 (4): 531–538.

Hale, T. W. 2012. *Medications and Mothers' Milk*. 15th ed. Amarillo, TX: Pharmasoft Medical Publishing.

Herbenick, D., et al. 2009. "Association of lubricant use with women's sexual pleasure, sexual satisfaction and genital symptoms: A prospective daily diary study." *Journal of Sexual Medicine* 6: 1867–1874.

Ip, S., et al. April 2007. *Breastfeeding and Maternal and Infant Health Outcomes in Developed Countries*. Evidence Report/Technology Assessment No. 153 AHRQ Publication No. 07-E007. Rockville, MD: Agency for Healthcare Research and Quality.

Leeman, L., et al. 2012. "Sex after Childbirth: Postpartum Sexual Function." *Obstetrics and Gynecology* 119 (3): 647–655.

Leitenberg, H., et al. 1995. "Sexual Fantasy." *Psychological Bulletin* 117 (3): 469–496.

Lentz, G., et al. 2012. *Comprehensive Gynecology*. 6th ed. Philadelphia, PA: Elsevier Publishing.

Light, K., et al. 2005. "More frequent partner hugs and higher oxytocin levels are linked to lower blood pressure and heart rate in premenopausal women." *Biological Psychology* 69 (1): 5–21.

Polomeno, V. 1999. "An Independent Study Continuing Education Program: Sex and Breastfeeding, An Educational Perspective." *Journal of Perinatal Education* 8 (1): 29–41.

Reader, F. 2005. "Is There Sex after Child Birth?" *Journal of the Association of Chartered Physiotherapists in Women's Health* 96: 35–40.

Roland, M., et al. 2005. "Breastfeeding and Sexuality Immediately Post-Partum." *Canadian Family Physician* 51: 1366–1367.

US National Library of Medicine. LactMed. http://toxnet.nlm.nih.gov/cgi-bin/sis/htmlgen?LACT.

Von Sydow, K. 1999. "Sexuality During Pregnancy and After Childbirth: A Metacontent Analysis of 39 Studies." *Journal of Psychosomatic Research* 47 (1): 27–49.

Von Sydow, K. 2002. "Sexual Enjoyment and Orgasm Postpartum: Sex Differences and Perceptual Accuracy Concerning Partners' Sexual Experience." *Journal of Psychosomatic Obstetrics and Gynecology* 23: 147–155.